HISTAMINE INTOLERANCE
EXPLAINED

- **SUPPLEMENTS**
- **DIET**
- **TIPS**

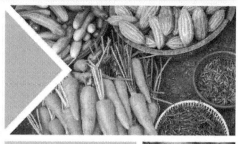

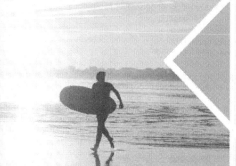

FOR A
**HEALTHY,
LOW-
HISTAMINE**
LIFE

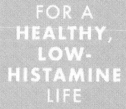

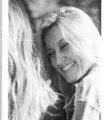

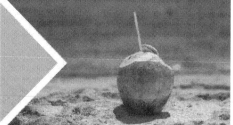

BY **KETOKO GUIDES**

HISTAMINE INTOLERANCE EXPLAINED

12 Steps To Building a Healthy Low Histamine Lifestyle

KETOKO GUIDES

Histamine Intolerance Explained: 12 Steps To Building a Healthy Low Histamine Lifestyle

TABLE OF CONTENTS

A PERSONAL STORY OF HISTAMINE INTOLERANCE

<u>It all started when…</u>

I suffered with digestive problems for 25 years, before I learnt the information that you are now going to read in this book. It all started when I was 18. Having previously been very healthy, I started to develop gut and digestive problems. Not so bad that I was in hospital, but bad in that I'd feel low energy the day after a few drinks with my buddies, eating a pizza, or sometimes just for seemingly no reason at all. Over the course of decades it got worse. The random gut pain, the inflammation, the dodgy back, the achy knees, the itchy skin, the headaches, and having a few days at a time when I felt lethargic, sick, anxious and low. The ups and downs seemed to get more and more random.

I tried a number of different diets, but nothing could make it any better. For days and sometimes weeks at a time, it would be absolutely fine. And then I would feel dreadful for no apparent reason. I'm guessing, since you've bought this book that a lot of this might resonate with you? If so, read on.

I tried everything – different exclusion diets, giving up certain foods, searching the internet, but nothing seemed to work. For sure, there were certain things that seemed to help. Giving up gluten was one. Whenever I went out and ate pizza or drank beer, my gut seemed to be a lot worse the next day. But it wasn't just that. Sometimes I would just head off to my local healthy café, eat some overpriced but delicious vegan burger that ticked all the right 'healthy' boxes, and the next day, boom, my symptoms were back, my gut was in pieces and I was back to square one. I just couldn't figure it out.

Getting worse

Over the course of those two decades or so, other symptoms started appearing as well. Blocked sinuses, runny eyes, bad hay fever, and achy and inflamed limbs. My knee was sometimes very sore and the next day not sore at all, I couldn't work out why. Hives, small itchy inflamed bumps on my hands and feet, especially in summer, what was that all about? And then more recently, I had headaches tingling on my forehead and severe fatigue. This really started to worry me. There was also an intolerance to alcohol, which got worse over time. Don't get me wrong, in my 20's and 30's I was drinking a lot. And that's probably going to hurt anyone's gut. But as time went on, I really seemed to develop quite an aversion to alcohol, especially red wine. There was one time when I was at a sporting event with friends. I probably only had three drinks, and they had a lot more so it was hardly like I was the big drinker of the group.

As the day wore on, I started to feel dreadful. Midway through the afternoon I had to make my excuses and head home. I managed to hail a taxi, but as we drew up outside my apartment I could barely get out of the car. I had to lie on the ground, I felt so bad. Eventually, I managed to crawl up my flat. I wanted to be sick but I couldn't. I felt so awful; it was like my stomach wanted to explode. What was going on?

I had only had a couple of drinks, and even felt like I'd been boring because I drank so little. And yet, my stomach was in pieces. What was going on?

What was going on was histamine intolerance.

Dr. Google doesn't have all the answers

In my searches across the internet, and in my consultations with doctors, I had seen and tried so many theories. Dr. Google never seemed to help. I had tried giving up meat, giving up gluten, giving up alcohol, giving up dairy, giving up carbs, giving up coffee, giving up virtually everything. I had read one or two doctors talking about histamine intolerance, but it seemed such a confusing and odd concept, that I didn't pay it much attention. Besides, all the websites on histamine intolerance seemed to contradict each other – confusing.

I didn't even really understand what histamine was all about. How could that apply to me? Eventually, having tried everything else (and I mean everything else), I started to look into histamine intolerance a little bit more. Hmmm. It was a diet that didn't massively appeal. Giving up red wine, avocado, leftovers, chocolate – hang on a sec, I like all those things. I thought I would give it a go.

The first signs of improvement

Wow. Not really knowing what I was doing, I started to follow a rudimentary low-histamine diet (you'll be doing this later in the book). I could say that I started to feel better within days, but honestly I started to feel better within hours.

The first thing to improve was my eyes became less watery. Oh yes, did I tell you I had watery eyes as one of my histamine symptoms? It may sound like a small symptom, but when your eyes are watering all the time, it's bloody annoying. It looks like you're crying or shedding tears, which isn't always a great look.

As it went on, my sinuses began to improve. And the really big thing for me – my digestive problem cleared up. It is no exaggeration to say that since the day I went on to a low-histamine lifestyle, my gut hasn't been quite as bad as it was previously. I've not had one gut flare up which was as bad as those I had in the dog days of my high-histamine life.

I knew when my gut was bad, it meant my energy levels were very low. It was hard to drag myself out of bed, let alone go about the important business of the day. So, to have such a dramatic improvement so quickly was amazing.

My nose cleared up, my digestion improved, the hives got better, the hay fever went down, and I felt way more energized, focused and healthy. All this happened quite quickly, but something it's important to remember is that it wasn't a linear improvement. Some days I was flying, and some days were low when my 'histamine bucket' overflowed. More on the bucket later. The point was though, that I was on the mend, and the impact on my overall health and energy was perhaps subtle to others, but genuinely life changing. And this was before I'd even got involved with some of the supplements and lifestyle practices you'll find in this book.

Tracking it to the next level

As you'll read in this book, there are different ways of measuring histamine intolerance. One of those that many overlook is through heart rate. For me, this has been massive and we'll go through it properly as we go on.

Affordable health tech is improving quickly. You can now buy very affordable heart rate trackers, sometimes a wristwatch or a ring that you wear and it measures your heartbeat. It may be moment-to-moment or just overnight depending on the tracker you purchase. I found the moment I started giving up histamine-rich foods, taking histamine supplements and living a low-histamine lifestyle, my heart rate lowered and my heart rate variability got higher. Even more excitingly, I could tell from day to day what food I ate and where my heart rate was at. In a nutshell, I could tell which foods I reacted to.

Do you realize how exciting this is? Histamine intolerance is notoriously hard to test, but as you read on, I'm going to outline the exact way in which you can track your own histamine levels 24/7, and start to work out your own personalized plan for what works. Because everyone is different, and that's why the low histamine food lists vary so wildly online. This is one of the 'secret sauce' moments in this book.

The Low Histamine Secret Sauce

Yes, we've sprinkled a number of 'secret sauce moments' throughout our guide. What does that mean? As you read on, you'll encounter a number of special low histamine tips that you may not read elsewhere, but have helped us hugely in our journey. And since us low histamine folk sometimes feel we aren't allowed a lot of the most delicious sauces, we've called it the Low Histamine Secret Sauce. Yum. Look out for this sign:

Low Histamine Secret Sauce!

We're going to build your own personalized histamine recovery plan, so read on to find out how to get saucy with your low histamine secret sauce.

Something to inspire you

This story is here to inspire you. As you read through this book, you may be in a place at the moment, where you feel very low physically and mentally. I hope this book helps lower your histamine bucket, improve your symptoms and take you to a healthier place. I hope it serves as an inspiration with 12 easy-to-read chapters. You might find that this information helps you going forward as well, as you read through this book. Understanding histamine has been a massive win for me, and I hope it will be for you as well.

You can read this book cover to cover, or simply consult the parts that you need most. Remember to take the quiz to see if you are histamine intolerant yourself.

Living with histamine intolerance can be frustrating, with conflicting advice on the best way to deal with this misunderstood condition. As far as possible, we have tried to cut through the confusion in this book, and present to you the best information that we have available.

If you are suffering now

If you're currently suffering from a severe attack of histamine induced

symptoms, please turn straight away to the chapter – 5 ways to reduce my histamine bucket right now!

We've written this chapter specifically for those who need help now. Unfortunately there is no 'magic pill' for reducing your histamine overload, but over the years of living with this condition, we have learnt simple solutions that quickly ease our symptoms.

<u>Getting more help</u>

Of course, this book is no substitute for consulting a medical practitioner. In fact, I highly recommend that you do so – and I have as part of my journey. You need to consult a professional medical practitioner, in order to ensure you are both able and healthy enough to participate in any suggestions in this book.

I highly recommend also consulting a functional health practitioner. You want to find somebody who will sympathetically listen to all your symptoms, your lifestyle factors, and the ways that you are affected by this condition. What's the point of this? Well it is to come up with a holistic, wide-ranging program for you to follow and to get better quickly.

It is possible. You can do it, with the help of this guide, the low histamine community (yes there is a community!) and expert practitioners. Across the 12 chapters, we'll help you every step of the way.

Good luck – let's get started!

Chapter 1

WHAT EVEN IS HISTAMINE INTOLERANCE?

Explaining a confusing condition – the technical bit

To understand histamine intolerance, we first need to first look at what histamine is. Now the following may get a bit technical, and feel free to move swiftly past this bit if you need help, like, now. But it's useful to understand a little bit more about what histamine does.

Okay, so, (deep breath), histamine is a chemical found in the body. It wears many hats. For one, it is helpful to the immune system, the central nervous system, and digestion (remember we were talking about digestion in the introduction). It equally doubles up as a neurotransmitter hence transports information to the brain. In digestion, it helps to break down food particles.

People going through histamine intolerance often have a deficiency of two vital enzymes in the body – diamine oxidase and histamine-N-methyltransferase. These are the primary enzymes that ensure a proper and controlled flow of histamine in the body. Without the two, then histamine build-up may be inevitable. Conversely, the symptoms will begin to appear.

If you have recently been a victim of any allergic reaction, you might have noticed the doctor prescribing some antihistamine meds. This is because histamine plays a role in these allergies. It causes inflammation to alert a person of a problem.

The swelling or dilation of blood vessels is as a result of histamine intervention (that's where the blocked nose comes in). This is a typical body mechanism, and the enzymes present will help to prevent any further build-up. So, if you are unable to break down histamine, due to some reasons, then this is what is referred to, medically, as histamine intolerance.

What's actually going on?

Histamine intolerance is the rapid increase of histamine in the body to uncontrollable levels. Since it traverses the entire body, histamine can affect several vital organs. For instance, it can cause damages to the cardiovascular system, the lungs, gut, skin, and central nervous system. This may result in several symptoms, which we will discuss in the subsequent chapter.

Now you're seeing why we need to sort all this out.

Contrary to what you might think, histamine intolerance does not mean sensitivity to histamine. It also doesn't imply an allergic reaction per se. It is only an indication that you have developed too much of this chemical in the body. Histamine hampers normal body processes and functions when it goes overboard. That's probably why you've bought this book. However, this doesn't imply that you don't want any histamine at all. It is supposed to exist in optimum amounts that neither damage the body nor affect sensitivity and processes. It's like a delicate balancing act.

The Dao Of Life

As much as it is not an allergic reaction, histamine is linked with the body's allergic responses. As mentioned above, there are two essential enzymes needed for histamine performance. One of them, known as diamine oxidase, or otherwise abbreviated as DAO, is affected by the following:

- Foods. Some foods block its performance and thus, affect the release of histamine. Other foods may also lead to abnormal functioning of the enzyme.

- Medications. Unfortunately, some meds may inhibit the production of this enzyme and thus, affect the performance of histamine.

- Disorders. Such as the gastrointestinal conditions e.g., inflammatory bowel syndrome and leaky gut syndrome.

The growth of bacteria can equally be the reason why you're histamine intolerant. So, you would wonder, how do I even get the bacteria in the first place? After all, if you're careful enough about your health and sanitation, it is almost impossible to get bacteria directly through eating. However, most of the bacteria in question comes from the improper digestion of food. This is what leads to high levels of histamine in the body.

In this instance, if you have average levels of DAO enzymes present, you cannot easily break down the histamine, which has skyrocketed. And this leads to a reaction in your body. The bucket is starting to overflow. It may be in the form of swelling and other symptoms. Oh, and just while we are on this point, inflammation, in particular, isn't necessary harmful. The only time it becomes a cause of concern, is when it becomes chronic. Inflammation is a perfectly natural bodily response. It's just when we have histamine intolerance, we can get too much of it.

It's important to note that when you're finally diagnosed with this condition, it's not like your life will never be the same. It merely means that you will need to adjust a few things in your life that may not go well with histamine. This includes looking at certain supplements, a lifestyle change and transforming your diet. Of course, we have this covered later on in the book.

More important technical stuff

Histamines are useful in the body and perform different functions, with the help of binding receptors. These receptors are spread throughout the body. And this is why you may notice that histamine symptoms go all over the body, from the head to the abdomen. The following is a brief list of the receptors related to histamine functioning, and their respective roles:

- **H1 receptors.** These are found all over the human body and result in the vasodilation of vessels.

- **H2 receptors.** Found in the stomach, they help in the release of stomach acid and increase the heart rate.

- **H3 receptors.** These are one of the sensitive ones because they are found inside the brain. They help in the coordination of nerves, appetite and sleeping. So, when next you cannot sleep nor eat, you know what to blame.

- **H4 receptors.** Lastly, these are found in the colon and small intestines. They are the ones that contribute to the body's inflammatory response.

As you may have already noticed, histamine controls our entire body. Therefore, we cannot do without them. It is only their improper breakdown and degradation that leads to problems such as histamine intolerance. So, you might wonder, where do these tiny chemical molecules emanate from?

Histamines primarily come off the gut. Hmmm, remember the gut issues we spoke about in the introduction. They can also be ingested through the foods we eat every day. In most cases, they will get in to the body through food that has some sort of bacterial infestation. That is why to prevent this from happening, you will need to eat only fresh foods or those that come from the freezer, especially if you're histamine intolerant.

The importance of diet

It is not quite possible to determine the amount of histamine found in food, especially while at home. Which makes it a histamine guessing game for us lot! In the labs, though, this might be easier due to the availability of equipment. But let's face it, we don't have a laboratory in our kitchen. This might also be the reason for the numerous contradictory remarks on the internet about food groups to use.

There are three things that may help you determine the bacterial load in food:

- The length of time food has stayed out without refrigeration.

- Whether or not the food has fermented.

- The type of bacteria found in the food.

So, for the above cases, you should try and avoid foods that don't pass the set requirements. In brief, don't eat food that has either fermented or stayed out of the fridge.

There are also a few food groups that accelerate your histamine intolerance. We will look at them in the subsequent chapters. But for now, here are some of the food groups and types to look out for:

- Foods that have vinegar.

- Fermented foods and beverages, including alcoholic drinks.

- Cured meats.

- Soured foods.

- Dried fruits.

- Smoked fish. Should only be fresh from the water or freezer.

- Most of the citrus fruits.

- Nuts. Put special emphasis on peanuts and walnuts.

- Aged cheese. In fact all cheese.

- Leftovers. (Unless frozen straightaway.)

Also, some foods don't exactly contain histamine, but trigger the release of the chemical in the mast cells. They include;

- Alcohol

- Avocado

- Chocolate

- Cow's milk

- Bananas

- Nuts

- Pineapple

- Papaya

- Strawberries

- Shellfish

- Tomatoes

- And most artificial preservatives.

Yes, yes, we realise there's some really really delicious stuff on the above lists. What you want me to give up eating avocado, chocolate, red wine and strawberries?

Well yes, for a while. But not necessarily forever. And besides, think how much better you'll feel.

Conversely, there are certain foods that inhibit the operation of DAO enzyme. They include;

- Energy drinks,

- Tea

- Alcohol.

But why some foods and not others? Very good question. Why are strawberries and raspberries, for example, supposedly higher in histamine than raspberries? It's a minefield, and that's why histamine intolerance is so poorly understood.

Underlying factors

Although it is not quite easy to tell what caused your histamine intolerance problem, there are some predisposing and underlying factors that may contribute. All this can be directly related to your capacity to break down histamine, and the following section is important. The following are some of the most common ones that you need to monitor:

- **Candida overgrowth.** There is a "brother-like" relationship between histamine and fungi. Fungal infections such as candida, a microbiome member, can lead to histamine intolerance. Immediately the body realizes that you have this fungal growth, it tries to get rid of it by all means. And you do know that when the body decides it is war against a foreign substance, then you are also to suffer in due process.

- **A leaky gut.** This allows large and undigested food to get into your bloodstream. Before food gets into your bloodstream, it needs to be properly digested and broken down into tiny molecules. Therefore, when the food you eat suddenly gets into the system in this improper manner, it alarms your immunity to respond. And the resulting response is the inflammation of the intestines. The reason why this is dangerous and leads to the intolerance of histamine, is because it hampers the functioning of DAO enzyme. And this is what leads to the high load of histamine in the body.

- **Non-steroidal anti-inflammatory drugs.** Otherwise abbreviated as NSAID, these are drugs that contribute to the inflammatory process in your gut. And this also suppresses the production of DAO enzyme. To be more precise, aspirin has been found to cause a huge release of histamine from the mast cells, when used by an individual.

- **Gut related bacteria.** Not all of the bacteria in the gut causes problems – some are beneficial, while some result in different issues. Gut bacteria either increases or reduces histamine dominance in the body. In some cases, the bacteria may neutralize the presence of histamine in the body and maintain it at optimum levels, which is the best case to happen anyway.

- **Small intestine bacterial overgrowth.** Abbreviated as SIBO, this also leads to inflammation in the gut. It can also lower the production of DAO enzymes in the body. As you may already know, histamine occurs due to the breakdown of the amino acid known as histidine by bacteria in the gut. This is why any overgrowth in the body can shoot up the production of histamine. The biggest risk factor that is present for SIBO is the low presence of stomach acids.

- **Genetics.** This will be covered later on in the text in detail. But for now, you should also know that it has a role to play in terms of histamine intolerance. The ABPI and AOC1 genes to be more specific, are the main ones that relate to histamine production. The HNMT gene can also contribute to the production of HNMT enzyme and DAO. Methylation issues can also lead to histamine related symptoms. And methylation occurs due to homozygous mutation.

- **Irritable bowel syndrome.** Shortened as IBS, this is a condition that leads to the overproduction of mucosal mast cells – and these are what release histamine.

- **Nutrient deficiencies.** Either vitamins or minerals, your body needs nutrients to perform optimally. Conversely, your histamine production may be affected when you lack certain nutrients in the body – especially those engaged in the production of DAO enzyme. Vitamin B6 and Vitamin C are specifically important in the production of DAO enzyme.

And this is probably why you will see vitamin C supplements suggested later in the book. In regards to minerals, magnesium is equally very important – and also suggested in the book. It is a mineral that helps to boost DAO activity. Poor dieting causes most nutrient deficiencies. Therefore, try as much to get the right diet to use.

So, just how can you know if what you're going through is histamine intolerance? Of course, we have a detailed coverage of the signs and symptoms in the next chapter, so you can head on there to see what the red flags are.

<u>So what's to blame?</u>

As much as you may want to blame histamine for your woes, weirdly, it really isn't the enemy. Histamine only comes out as normal reflex responses to what you're going through at the moment. In fact, it comes to help, rather than causing harm. To inform your body that something isn't right. It is vital for numerous bodily processes including; the removal of toxins, the release of stomach acid and boosting the immune system.

It is quite right to state that histamines are never the enemy, until when they are either overproduced or when they can't be broken down properly. Infections, genetics and leaky gut are the best-known causative agents of histamine intolerance. Therefore, maintaining a healthy gut will be your most precious tool for warding off histamine intolerance.

The symptoms may be quite uncomfortable for you as an individual. And sometimes no one may understand the depth and intensity of your pains more than yourself – not even your doctor. However, if you feel that you might be going through the condition, it is vital for you to first seek advice from the doctor. Hopefully this guide can work alongside the expert assistance you receive.

Having understood what histamine intolerance is, we can now move forward to the next chapter. Do you have histamine intolerance? Let's find out.

Chapter 2

Do I have histamine intolerance?

Many people suffer the effects of histamine intolerance, which are let's be honest, not exactly fun. But it's hard to know if what you are going through is histamine intolerance, or something else? So let's find out.

The common symptoms that most people experience include severe headaches, digestive technicalities such as diarrhea, rhinitis, and eczema. Allergic rhinitis is what many know as hay fever. The more prevalent and potent symptoms encompass, asthma, and rapid heartbeat.

The general symptoms of histamine intolerance vary from one individual to the other. But here are some of the primary signs and symptoms that act as a wake-up call for this condition: We thought we'd put together a little histamine intolerance quiz. Take a look down the symptoms and see how many you've suffered from. Then compare your score at the end.

<u>Quiz</u>

Look through the below histamine-related symptoms, and make a note of how many apply to you.

- Gut issues. This may arise either after eating food or before. It may be gut pain, or bowel issues

- Diarrhea. This may be part of the abdominal pains you will encounter regularly or come on sporadically, or when your histamine bucket gets too full.

- Bloating. Too much gas from your abdomen may also be a sign of intolerance to histamine. However, this may not be a sure sign because it may also translate to something else. (This is why histamine intolerance is so confusing.)

- IBS. Irritable bowel syndrome.

- Nausea.

- Chronic constipation. This is no ordinary constipation that arises from fiber shortage in the diet. You may be taking fiber frequently but still, experience constipation to a high level.

- Inflammation. This is a really big one. Do you have a sore back/achy knees/bad wrist? Do your joints ache? Histamine can cause this.

- Anxiety. Since it affects the central nervous system, histamine intolerance can cause anxious thoughts and feelings. You will rarely know the reason why you're anxious. (This can really mess with our heads – and can be one of the best things about embarking on the program in this book.)

- Shortage of breath. Sometimes you may become short of breath. Yes, uneasy breathing is a sign of histamine intolerance

- Severe menstrual strain and pain. (Not the same as the regular cycle that occurs every month during the cycle. Only when it becomes unbearable, or becomes worse over time)

- A boosted heart rate at times. You notice your heart racing on occasions. Your heart beats beyond the regular palpitations and might even cause a heavy feeling on the chest.

- Any skin problems. This might include dry skin, eczema, and scaly or patchy skin.

- Hives are very common with histamine. Small red bumps anywhere on the skin. The skin may also become itchy.

- Exhaustion. You may experience an exhausted body and fail to understand why. Sometimes this occurs even when you had nothing much to do throughout the day.

- Dizziness. Once in a while, you may feel dizzy, or sleepy out of nowhere.

- Constant sneezes. This mostly occurs in the early hours of the night.

- Watery eyes. Your eyes may be teary, and this may not result from any 'normal' problem in particular. They may also turn red and become itchy from time to time.

- Running nose or blocked nose. An itchy sensation and a congested feeling may follow this.

- Headache. This may develop from mild feelings to severe cases where it becomes chronic.

- Sleeping disorders. You may encounter the inability to sleep, which may develop into insomnia. You might wake too early, or wake in the middle of the night, or find your sleep disrupted.

- Reduced blood pressure.

- Tremors and chills.

- Loss of consciousness.

Results

0 symptoms: Congratulations – it looks like you don't have histamine intolerance. But it doesn't completely rule it out, as you may be suffering other symptoms that we haven't covered in this book.

1 – 4 symptoms: You might have histamine intolerance. But the confusing thing about this condition is that the symptoms are so wide-ranging. The best thing to do is follow the program in the rest of this book, and see if you start to feel better. If you do then, you have histamine intolerance, and the great news is, you've found the solution too.

5 or more symptoms: The frustrating thing about histamine intolerance is it's tough

to test for it, and it's hard to get a diagnosis. However, based on your score, it's very possible you have histamine intolerance. Move straightaway to the practical steps in this book and see if you start to feel better.

Chapter 3

WHAT IS MY "HISTAMINE BUCKET"?

It's one of our favourite terms

The "histamine bucket" is a commonly used term in the low histamine community. Is there a 'low histamine community'? Supposedly there is. There certainly are plenty of people willing to offer help, support and love when you're going through the kind of symptoms that you might be going through now as you read this book.

The histamine bucket refers to a bucket that you might think of, that is filled up with your personal histamine levels. You can eat all of the wrong foods, do all of the wrong things in terms of histamine, and as long as your bucket doesn't overflow, you'll be alright. You might not notice your symptoms until the bucket overflows

When the bucket overflows

It might be that one bit of cheese or fermented food that tips you over the edge. It might be a glass of wine, a strawberry, or a peanut. Sometimes you won't know what it was. And when your bucket overflows, your symptoms start to come crashing in.

That's what we refer to as the histamine bucket.

You want to keep your bucket as empty as possible – your histamine bucket as low as possible. This is so those symptoms don't come crashing.

Emptying your bucket

The rest of the chapters in the book are all focused on keeping your histamine bucket as empty as possible, to keep you as symptom free as possible. And it's not just diet supplements, there's lifestyle as well – sleeping well, reducing your stress, doing exercise. All of these are so important. And not necessarily strenuous exercises every day. We like relaxed exercises like walking, yoga, breathing, and meditation. All of this good stuff can help empty the histamine bucket.

Your body, remember, requires histamine to do plenty of things. The ideal amount of histamine is perfect for you, but the problem for many of us is that we've got more than the ideal amount of histamine. As histamine levels go up, your intolerance levels can go up as well. And that's when problems start to occur. That's when the histamine bucket can start to spill over and overflow. You need to get rid of some of that fast. Read on to learn how to reduce your histamine bucket and empty some of it.

Consider it our mission to empty your bucket, and get you feeling a lot better.

Chapter 4

THE LOW-HISTAMINE DIET –
WHICH FOODS SHOULD I AVOID?

You may have already spent some time investigating histamine intolerance and diets. You may already have realised that it's an absolute minefield. One site says that something is absolutely fine, the next site says it's not. Take blueberries for example. Some say its okay, some say you will have a histamine attack – who to believe? (We are obsessed with frozen blueberries, and they don't seem to affect us, but you'll have to work out whether they affect you or not.)

There are so many conflicting food items in histamine intolerance. Beef, chocolate, cacao, and berries – all of these seem to conflict on the major sites. Let's try and make some sense of it here in this book.

There are, thankfully, certain foods that are almost universally acknowledged as a no, when it comes to histamine production. We're going to go over the main elements here, and we want to direct you to an incredible list online that we think is the conclusive resource when it comes to histamine and diet. The best histamine food list online (pdf) is published by the odd sounding *Swiss Interest Group Histamine Intolerance (SIGHI)* – the lengths some will go to get an acronym that makes sense eh. But we have a lot to thank SIGHI as their pdf is really helpful for us histamine intolerant folk. It's not perfect (none of these lists are), but you might want to bookmark their pdf or download it. We have. And then when you are out and about and need to check whether a particular food might or might not be high in histamine, you can check with SIGHI and they'll point you in the right direction.

In the meantime, here's more on some of the chief dietary histamine culprits.

Fermented foods

Definitely steer clear of these. The very way that they are created using bacteria means that's something that could increase your histamine bucket – you don't want that. Fermented foods include sauerkraut, kefir, kombucha and many others.

Avocados

Avocados, you are joking, right? We had always presumed that avocado was pretty much the healthiest food I could possibly eat. High and good fats, low in carbs and absolutely delicious at the same time. Use it in salads, eat it by itself, you can even make avocado cheesecake. But not if you're histamine intolerant, because, it is very unfair, isn't it? But avocados are out.

Chocolate

Unfortunately, histamine intolerance means that some of the most delicious foods out there are out. But don't worry, because once you lower your histamine bucket and empty out some of that bad stuff, it doesn't mean that you can never have these foods. Only that you start to have more control around them. And let's face it, if you feel great, that is a major incentive to avoid all these foods. We love all the foods on this list pretty much, but we love feeling good a lot more.

Chocolate is one of the items most people say you should avoid. Some say that cacao in its raw state seems to be okay in terms of histamine. They can't quite work out why cacao is okay but chocolate is not.

To us, that sounds dodgy and I think we should stick with the fact that cacao and chocolate is out. Sorry!

A good substitute to chocolate is carob and you can buy some delicious carob bars from your local health food store. However, wait for it, some sites say that carob is also high in histamine. As always, it's really important that you do your own research. Because this list will not be conclusive for everybody. For some people, they'll be fine with chocolate while for others, they won't be. Unfortunately, the only way to work it out is to test it yourself.

Fish

Most fresh organic, pasture-raised meats seem to be okay, but fish does seem to be high on histamine. It is something about how the bacteria grows in the fish, once it's being caught. If the fish is caught and frozen immediately, that can be better. But you'll find most fish appears on histamine banned lists. There are certain fish that are better than others. But for the most part, fish and histamine don't go together, and are not happy bed fellows.

Leftovers

Previously, there was nothing I used to love more than having a massive cook up on a Sunday, and then sorting out all my food for the week. Lots of lovely portions waiting for me in the fridge every morning. I didn't have to think about food until Friday. Unfortunately, that's out when it comes to histamine. Because leftovers increase in bacteria and histamine the more they've been left. There is a way round this and that is; when you cook your food and you'd like to eat leftovers afterwards, put them straight in the freezer compartment. When you're ready to eat, defrost thoroughly and then heat up, obviously within safety guidelines.

Citrus

For some reason, citrus is out. It seems unfair, doesn't it? So many delicious things on this list. But as always, test. If you are okay with citrus, then that's fine. You'll soon know once you start tuning in on what makes you intolerant and what doesn't.

Cheeses

Most cheeses are extremely high in bacteria and histamine, they have to be avoided. The same unfortunately goes for processed meats.

Alcohol

Alcohol and histamine don't seem to go together. It is such a shame it took me 25 years to work this out. If you do still fancy the odd drink though, all is not lost. Thankfully there are some alcohols that seem to work better than others.

First the ones to look out for. Red wine, and in fact, wines of all description, seem to be the worst. Yes that includes prosecco! And, if you remember the particular attack we told you about, the one when I went to the sporting event with my friends a while back, that was a red wine attack.

Thankfully since then, some of the wonderful people in the histamine community have offered some suggestions on how best to enjoy the odd glass of something alcoholic, and feel okay the next day. Be warned, we are just talking about a measured glass or two of something nice. Many suggested tequila, but I have found a certain clean vodka seems to work better than just about anything else. It's called Tito's vodka, and seems to be particular popular in the USA. Should I be recommending alcohol in a book about histamine? Well all the usual caveats about sensible drinking apply.

We are unfortunately Mr. and Mrs. Sensitive these days when it comes to booze. But just like many people, we still do want the very occasional drink. And we might have cracked it, with my new favorite vodka. The idea is, that the less impurities there are in an alcohol, the less likely you are to react to it. In other words, the less likely it is to give you a stinking histamine hangover.

Low Histamine Secret Sauce!

Okay, it's time for our first secret sauce alert. Tito's handmade vodka is micro distilled six times in an old-fashioned pot and is described as a spectacularly clean product of incomparable excellence. Only the heart, the nectar is taken. And the vodka is cleansed by filtering it through the finest activated carbon available. It doesn't seem to give me the night sweats after drinking it, so is worth a look.

By the way we have no affiliation with them. We should really get them to sponsor this book! That said, you might find you react to it, so really you just have to simply test gently and see whether you have a flare-up. If so, you can rule the vodka out in the interests of feeling histawesome.

In summary – histamine heavy foods

Broadly speaking you want to avoid

- Foods that have vinegar. (Apple Cider Vinegar might be okay)

- Fermented foods and beverages, including alcoholic drinks.

- Cured meats.

- Soured foods.

- Dried fruits.

- Smoked fish. Should only be fresh from the water or freezer.

- Most of the citrus fruits.

- Nuts. Put special emphasis on peanuts and walnuts.

- Aged cheese. In fact all cheese.

- Leftovers. (Unless frozen straightaway.)

- Eggs (for some people – particularly egg whites)

- Alcohol

- Avocado

- Chocolate

- Cow's milk

- Bananas

- Nuts

- Pineapple

- Papaya

- Strawberries

- Shellfish

- Tomatoes

- And most artificial preservatives.

- Energy drinks,

- Tea

- Alcohol.

The ketogenic and the low-carb diet

The ketogenic and low carb diets seems to work particularly well for all sorts of health issues. Increasingly in the natural health world, the importance of good fats is emphasized alongside reducing sugars and carbs. That means less white bread and ice cream, but more delicious olive oil, with butter and high-fat treats.

Both the ketogenic and the low-carb diet are similar, because they support a low carbohydrate intake. However, they are not entirely the same and may have a few differences. Both of them are an effective option for histamine intolerance. This is due to the healthy food options they encourage. Some individuals may thrive better in a low-carb diet than a ketogenic diet, and vice versa. In a nutshell, for both diets, the following foods are permitted and encouraged:

- **Fats** – for this group, you can take anything from butter, olive oil, egg yolks, coconut oil and milk, olive oil etc. It is important to only take the egg yolk, while avoiding the egg white (for some people – egg white is high histamine). Also, for butter, it shouldn't be cultured. Oh and we have found crème fraiche, while delicious, is high on the ol' histamine too.

- **Protein** – here you can eat poultry, fish (occasionally, as per the above lists), seafood and meat. Please note that everything **MUST** be very fresh or frozen, especially when it comes to seafood.

- **Nuts and seeds** – for this group, you are restricted from any other nuts and seeds, except chia and macadamia. But test, because you might react okay. Some lists say nuts are absolutely fine, but we've found them to provoke histamine issues.

- **Vegetables** – yes please, great for keto and low-carb, great (often) for low-histamine, essential in the body for the great nutrients and benefits. Some of the examples encouraged include beets, asparagus, artichoke, cauliflower, carrot, cabbage, fennel, cucumber, celery, lettuce, green beans, nettle, radishes, white onion and zucchini. Sadly not tomatoes.

- **Fruits** – this group also plays a huge role in the body. Examples include coconut, apple, figs, mango, kiwi, pear, melon, pomegranate, persimmon and star fruit. Be cautious with raspberries, strawberries and pineapple.

- **Beverages** – aside from water, try and limit yourself to rooibos tea, nettle tea and peppermint tea. Oh and coffee. We love coffee. So much. Make mine a Flat White with coconut milk. Most lists have coffee as fine for low-histamine, but again you need to check your own personal sensitivity.

<u>Why keto?</u>

Over 20 studies made on the ketogenic diet alone have shown its benefits and contributions towards good health – especially for histamine intolerant patients. The problem is that with the added introduction of histamine, you have to work a little harder to make keto work. But it's still possible. Why is it such a good idea?

The reduction of carbs in the ketogenic diet allows for a state known as ketosis to come into place. This makes your body extra efficient and fast in burning fat, which is helpful in preventing different ailments. In the liver, your fats turn into ketones. It is this ketones that improve brain functionality and it is the brain that controls the metabolic processes that take place in the body. Therefore, when it is functioning optimally, this results in the smooth functioning of all bodily processes, including histamine production. Interesting bit: Your histamine production may sky-rocket when your brain is not correctly controlling metabolism.

The ketogenic diet advises you to cut down on sugars, pastries, soda, alcohol and other junk. Which is effective not just for histamine intolerant patients, but also for everyone. Junk foods and drinks have excessive calories and insufficient nutrients, or none at all – this is harmful for all of us on a prolonged basis. It takes around three to four days on this diet, before your body starts to burn protein and fat. This is due to the absence of carbs, which act as the typical fuel source in the body. There are different types of ketogenic diet, and you should choose one that you are most comfortable with. Some of the most common examples include the following:

- **The standard ketogenic diet.** It is the most common variant used by most individuals. It is very low in carbohydrates, moderate in protein and very high in fat. Typically, you would expect to take 75% of fat, 20% of protein and 5% of carbs.

- **Cyclical ketogenic diet.** Here, you will have certain periods where you will take higher carb refeeds. So, it is more like an intermittent ketogenic diet, where you have 5 days of intensive ketogenic diet, followed by 2 days of high carbohydrate intake.

- **Targeted ketogenic diet.** With this diet, you only add carbs to your meals when working out. This helps to give your body sufficient energy to go over the entire process.

- **High protein ketogenic diet.** The only difference between this diet and the standard ketogenic variant is that it includes more protein. For instance, you can expect a ratio like 60% fats, 35% protein and 5% of carbs.

It is advisable to follow the standard ketogenic diet and the high protein ketogenic diet, as the other ones lack sufficient study to prove their effectiveness. The standard ketogenic diet is specifically the best to use since it does not strain you a lot, especially as a beginner. Remember, you are not using the ketogenic diet for weight loss purposes. You are using it to boost your health and immunity.

Having looked at the foods permitted in the ketogenic diet; you might start to think how boring it really is. However, there are some amazing snacks that you can still eat. Yes, snacks that will satisfy your taste buds, but still keep your health in check. You will still need to observe caution with how much you eat. One of the things we found useful with keto was to batch cook, then save smaller portions of leftovers in the freezer.

It is equally a diet that is not easy to eat out with. You can easily get good options when visiting a friend or restaurant. However, more and more restaurants are beginning to incorporate histamine friendly foods in their menus, and in this case, the ketogenic diet. Also, if you are unable to eat the ketogenic foods, there are various supplements that you can use instead. Some of them include the following:

- **Exogenous ketones.** Such supplements help to raise the levels of ketones in the body. As earlier stated, this helps the brain to fasten metabolic processes.

- **MCT oil.** This is added to different drinks such as yoghurt and helps to boost ketone levels. It may also be useful in boosting your energy levels, especially when you feel worn out by the histamine symptoms. You can get great options and variants of this oil online, through stores like amazon. Should be fine with histamine.

- **Creatine.** This supplement has various uses and benefits in terms of performance and health. It is particularly great if you are using it alongside the ketogenic diet and exercises.

- **Caffeine.** Did we say we love coffee? Check on your histamine and coffee relationship but most of the food lists around approve.

- **Minerals.** Mineral supplements help in many ways, especially for salt and magnesium, which we will look at later on. They are particularly great as a beginner in the diet, because they help to regulate shifts in water. We take magnesium chloride supplements every evening, in spray and liquid form, and find it helps also with sleep.

Similar to every other thing on the planet, the ketogenic diet isn't perfect. And so, it has a number of disadvantages and side effects – which we must let you know. But prior to that, we need to learn more about ketosis and how you would know when in this state. This is the main process in the diet, that advocates for its health benefits in the body. In the context of histamine, you have to work out if it's actually helping your histamine health. Here are some of the ways you will know when you're in ketosis, which are equally the ways to know if the diet is working for you or not:

- **Weight loss.** Keeping your weight in check is no loss at all. Even if you intended to only boost your health and prevent the dominance of histamine, you can consider this as a win-win situation. Therefore, when in ketosis, it would make perfect sense if you lose some weight. In case this doesn't happen, you should be concerned. However, the ketogenic diet is not a magic pill, and so, don't expect this sign to come immediately. In fact, you may even gain weight in the initial stages. Until when you get to ketosis, you will probably maintain your current weight. Besides, what you witness as weight loss within the first few days of the diet should not deceive you, as this is simply water weight. The real weight that will be lost after several weeks is the fat weight.

- **Thirst.** Are you feeling thirsty more often after starting the keto diet? Yes, that's probably due to ketosis. This process may make you to feel a bit thirstier than normal. And this is mostly an effect of water loss in the body. A good practice, therefore, would be to take water constantly, and take a small pinch of Himalayan salt in your water at times. Be careful not to get into dehydration as this may complicate the process, and make things worse not better.

- **Boosted levels of ketones.** As earlier pointed out, the ketosis process leads to the production of an important fuel for the brain and body – ketones. To check for ketone levels in the blood, doctors might need to take a urine sample from you or conduct breath tests. The most reliable tests, however, are the blood tests. You can equally use a specialized home kit to measure these levels and see whether or not they are present. On average, you should register 0.5-3 millimoles per liter of ketones in your body if you are in ketosis. These testing kits can easily be bought online.

- **Muscle spasms and cramps.** These effects usually arise due to the electrolyte imbalance and the dehydration process in the body as detailed above. In case you didn't know this; electrolytes carry electrical signals between different body cells. Therefore, when they are interrupted or imbalanced, this leads to disruptions in the transmission of electric messages. This is what leads to twitching and cramping of the muscles. To replenish electrolytes, take sufficient water and good quality salt.

- **Headaches.** Be careful not to mistake this for a histamine intolerance symptom. Uh, maybe that's why it is hard to diagnose histamine. Back to the current subject, headaches may arise when you get into ketosis. They occur due to the deficiency of carbohydrates and sugar in your body. Also, they can arise due to electrolyte imbalances and dehydration. Oh yes, dehydration is becoming a theme. Makes perfect sense and that is why you will always get a persistent headache when you don't take enough water. The interesting bit of it all is that ketosis is ultimately a cure for headaches and migraines. Funny eh?

- **General body fatigue.** This may be followed by body weakness. However, it is a common sign in the initial stage of ketosis and fades away later on. Mostly, this arises due to the change of fuel from carbohydrates to fats. And dehydration. We're sounding like a broken record now. Rehydrate. It's more than that though. You will notice the difference because carbs have a quicker burst of energy for the body when compared to the fats. After several weeks of ketosis, your body will then adapt to the new fuel source, and you will begin to notice an increased energy level.

- **Stomach aches.** This can also be confusing as it is a common sign for histamine intolerance as well. But you should note that any slight change of diet is bound to cause you some upsets in the stomach. This may also be accompanied with other digestive complications. The ketogenic diet, and ketosis to be more specific, is no exception. You are likely to face the same challenges in this diet. Water intake and other fluids may help to ease this problem. Besides, you will also need to take non-starchy vegetables, together with other fiber-filled delicacies to help you reduce constipation. For a healthier gut, you can also consider taking a probiotic supplement. We like ProBiota HistaminX by Seeking Health as it's histamine friendly. More on supplements coming later.

- **Sleeping variations and disorders.** Once you're in ketosis, this might be inevitable. You may start to experience difficulty sleeping. However, this should go away within a few weeks. It's your body adapting to a new food source.

- **Foul smelling breath.** This is one of the common signs you will notice when in ketosis. This is because the ketones inside your body leave through urine and breath. A specific type of ketone known as acetone is the main responsible for the bad smell. Others that may also contribute include acetophenone and benzophenone. There is no sure way of alleviating this issue. However, it tends to reduce with time. You can use breath fresheners to reduce the stench. Most sugar gums flavoured with xylitol are fine although tend to have 1g of sugar. Always always avoid aspartame in chewing gum and everywhere else.

- **Boosted focus and concentration.** This is another positive effect of ketosis. Those who have tried out the diet report a better and boosted mental clarity and concentration.

So, having seen what to look out for when trying to learn if you're in ketosis or not, let us now see what the side effects of the ketogenic diet are – take a look below:

- A keto flu.

- Boosted hunger.

- Insomnia.

- Nausea.

- Digestive errors, though limited.

- Decreased performance in exercises, in some cases.

- Nausea.

- Water and mineral imbalance.

Don't let this put you off though – the low carb or ketogenic diet may not work for everyone but it's really worth considering alongside your histamine issues as it can help to heal your gut – by reducing the sugar and the bacteria in there.

Keto or low-carb? What to do?

If ketosis seems too much, perhaps consider using the low-carb diet. But just what does the low-carb diet entail?

First, you need to know that the low carb diet, just as the name, is low in carbohydrates. Duh. Instead, you feed on other macros such as fats and proteins. You also have the option of adding veggies to the mix if you can. Studies have shown the various health benefits of low-carb diets. They have been in existence for a long time, and have gotten the approval of many dieticians and medical practitioners. The best part about this diet is that, unlike other diets, there is no need to use special products or online calculators and trackers.

This diet is safe for most individuals. However, it is advisable that you don't start or seek further advice if you fall under the following category:

- Breastfeeding.

- Taking medications.

If you don't fall under the above groups, you're okay to start the diet. But for those taking meds, you can seek counsel from your doctor to see if you may be able to handle the diet. Some medications will work perfectly with a low carb diet. For instance, most histamine-related meds don't have a problem in regards to the low carb diet.

Happy gut

One of the reasons we love the low carb diet is because it is friendly to the gut. This is a sensitive part in the body that easily gets affected by the effects of histamine intolerance. The low carb diet might be very helpful in cooling down a grumpy and painful gut. Aside from the irritable bowel syndrome, it also helps to reduce bloating and severe gut pains. In addition, it is good at clearing diarrhea and gas, something you might know too much about with your histamine issues. If you have reflux, indigestion and any other digestive abnormalities, this may equally improve when you use the low carb diet. Those who have experienced the severity of histamine symptoms acknowledge that this is one of the best reasons to use the low carb diet.

Starting a low carb diet is not a walk in the park, but can make you feel really great, and you may be surprised at how quickly your energy levels increase and your capacity to deal with histamine issues improves. NB – you may notice reduced tolerance to alcohol. Well, this isn't really a bad effect if you are looking to reduce your histamine bucket.

A low carb diet can work really well for you, based on how you use it. You can gain numerous benefits and this can help your immunity improve, especially for histamine intolerant cases. However, you can easily miss out on all this if you get low-carb wrong.

- **Eating too little portions of carbs.** It is a low carb diet, and not a no carb diet. This is where most people go wrong on the diet. You are only supposed to reduce the amount of carbs you take and not totally get rid of them. It is so easy for you to suffer a carb crash when you are taking in extremely low bits of carbs. And this is why you may start to give up on the diet right before you advance. All the macros need to be present in your meal plan. You're going for low-carb not keto here.

- **Skiving greens.** Veggies are very important in any diet. And if you find any meal plan that excludes them, then it is not the right one to use. As much as dieticians may argue that fruits and greens are filled with carbs, the fact remains that you cannot do without them. After all, since it is a low carb diet, you can make sure that the most carbs you take fall under the fruits and vegetables group. The standard rule is that your plate should either be full of greens or half full. And you can drizzle loads of good olive oil on top.

- **Evading fiber.** This is a vital nutrient that helps to curb gastrointestinal disturbances, most of which occur due to constipation. You get sufficient roughages from the greens you eat. When you start cutting out carbs, you may also tend to experience bloating, which you can highly reduce through the consumption of dietary fiber.

- **Failure to plan.** You need to have a proper plan before starting anything, quite literally. And a diet is no exception, as failing to plan might lead you into dropping out just as you have started. So, you need to think ahead on what you will eat for example. Since there are certain rules to be followed, you will need to consider what options you choose, so that they fall under the permitted category.

- **Failure to exercise.** As much as you may tend to dismiss this, it is very essential when you're in a diet. This is to help the body burn fuel even more.

<u>Conclusion</u>

As you can see, we have done an in-depth analysis of both diets, to give you an easier time when deciding which one to use. You can also interchange both of them to see which one suits you most.

Ultimately, both the keto and the low-carb diets are a little bit tougher when you have to think about histamine too, but it's perfectly doable and many people who live with histamine intolerance do exactly this – finding that a low-carb approach helps them manage their symptoms even better. Alongside your new diet, perhaps you can use some supplements to boost your nutrition intake. Take a look at some of the best to use in the subsequent chapter.

Chapter 5

THE BEST LOW-HISTAMINE SUPPLEMENTS

The symptoms of histamine intolerance are often similar to allergies, but more pronounced. All of these symptoms, from watery/itchy eyes to sneezing, congestion and sinus problems can soon become very uncomfortable and unbearable. When you add all the other issues we mentioned in the previous chapter, you might be tempted to opt for over the counter medications.

We are not against these necessarily, but would always prefer a natural approach first up.

As much as some pharmaceutical approaches may work in your favor, they may leave you with a trail of painful side effects, especially in the long run.

<u>Naturally speaking</u>

Understanding how histamine works is the trick to getting the best natural supplements to keep you going. We have had some great success with the supplements listed below, so let us guide you through some of the best ways to reduce your histamine overload and get happy, healthy and fit. And once you've looked through the supplements, make sure you check out the 'meditation not medication' section, which might be the most important in the book.

ProBiota HistaminX

ProBiota HistaminX is an excellent supplement from one of our favourite practitioners Dr. Ben Lynch. Incidentally he has some great online resources based on the relationship with histamine and genetics.

His company Seeking Health created this supplement aims at supporting the body's healthy digestion and microbiome. They created it because many probiotics can cause more harm than good for histamine. This one though contains entirely histamine-friendly strains of bacteria.

It may also aid in boosting the metabolism of histamine taken into the body. ProBiota HistaminX contains probiotics that are safe for the gut and reduce histamine rather can causing a flare up. It helps to reduce the histamine-producing bacteria, and is best to take after your dinner. We like taking it last thing at night. Also, it needs to be kept away from harmful microbials. Some bacterial species produce histamine, while others are essential in breaking it down.

Here are some of the benefits of this supplement:

- It is ideal for both vegans and meat lovers.

- Helps to tune the gut's response to the ingested histamine.

- Boosts the immunity of a person.

- Helps to enhance the gut microbiome.

- Has histamine-friendly probiotics that won't cause a flare up in your gut.

All in all, we give this supplement a 10 out of 10 for histamine.

HistaminX

HistaminX is another great supplement from Dr. Ben Lynch's company. It has both herbal and plant-derived compounds that work together to ease inflammation and histamine effects. It is often argued that changes in diets and environment spike different allergies in the body. This supplement helps to prevent these changes from increasing your histamine bucket.

HistaminX is a supplement that also helps to tone down those seasonal allergies that keep on reoccurring. In addition, it prevents the blunt histamine symptoms from draining you.

Unless otherwise directed by your doctor, it is best to take this supplement in the afternoon and evening (always read the label and follow the instructions). Besides, you can equally take it when you feel the attack from histamine symptoms. This will help to relieve the pains you are going through.

If you are not having histamine symptoms, you might want to avoid taking the supplement totally, or otherwise take it once in a day. It is a great reliever of running nose, congestion and many other allergies. As it is fairly new in the market, you should use it alongside medical advice.

Here are some of its benefits:

- Supports the body's healthy and healing process.

- Ideal for both meat lovers and vegans.

- Boosts immune health and well-being.

- Brings about seasonal comfort to the body.

- Supports healthy mucoid membranes. This may be of great help in terms of sinuses and congestion.

We like this supplement a lot and give it 8 out of 10.

Quercetin

This is one of our very favourites, and stand by for a secret sauce moment coming up. We like BioCare's Quercetin Plus for the purity and, well, it just seems to work well.

Aside from being a supplement, Quercetin is a compound found in several plants. It is an antioxidant that exists naturally in apples and onions, among many other foods. But you'd have to eat a lot of onions to get the amount found in a supplement. Research-based findings have led to the release of supplements like BioCare containing this compound, due to its antihistamine effects. Depending on your choices or preferences, you can either buy quercetin-rich food (onion-breath alert) or head for the supplements. As one of the most trusted mast cell stabilizers, quercetin is a potent antioxidant. This supplement controls the mast cells from releasing histamine. As it takes time to be absorbed in the body, many brands recommend it is taken at least 15-30 minutes before your meal.

Here are some of its benefits:

- Reduces allergic symptoms.

- Helps support the body's ability to quench free radicals

- Reduces inflammatory response that may lead to allergic reactions.

- Reduces respiratory side effects.

- Can help with the side effects of dust, pollen, hay fever and sun.

- Helps with prostate symptoms.

- Is thought to help prevent cancer cell growth in breast, colon, prostate, endometrial and lung.

Low Histamine Secret Sauce!

We found when we started to take one BioCare Quercetin tablet in the middle of the night, our sleep dramatically improved. It may sound odd, but we were waking up early every morning and couldn't work out why. With this, once we took the Quercetin in the middle of the night, we slept like a baby. It's a massive change. Please consult your doctor before using this approach as it may not be recommended for you personally. Always check with your healthcare provider before starting new supplements or protocols. However Quercetin really works for us.

We give Quercetin 10 out of 10.

Pycnogenol

Tree bark. Amazing innit. This is an extract of the bark of the Pinus Pinaster, otherwise known as French Maritime Tree Bark. Pycnogenol has a potency to fight free radicals in the body. These are by-products of metabolism that are normal in the body, but harmful when in large portions.

Low Histamine Secret Sauce!

Pycnogenol inhibits the release of histamine from the mast cells in the body, and it's often overlooked in the fight against an allergic response. Not here though – it's one of our secret sauce moments. Here are some of its benefits:

- Reduces allergy symptoms and inflammation.

- Wards off free radicals in the body.

- Prevents the release of histamine from mast cells.

- Helps to relieve circulation problems.

- We regularly use this and give it 7.5 out of 10.

Colostrum

This is a type of milk produced by cows (oh and humans), a few days after giving birth. We recommend the Surthrival brand and have had great success using it. Just to be clear – this is cow colostrum not human colostrum, and you always want to use a brand where the newborn have their share of the milk before the supplement is made.

Why is it so good? Colostrum is rich in antibodies. These antibodies help to boost an individual's immune system. Aside from histamine intolerance, it is popularly used to correct several other complications in the body. Here are some of its known benefits:

- Helps to prevent allergic reactions.

- Ideal for fat burning.

- Helps to ease gastrointestinal challenges.

- Eases diarrhea caused by infections and allergies.

- Suppresses histamine dominance.

- We give this supplement 8.5 out of 10.

Grass fed kidney for DAO

Grass-fed kidney is an excellent source of DAO, but let's face it, who has the time to cook up a load of kidney every day, and then eat it fresh so it doesn't accumulate histamine in the fridge? DAO, as you now know, is a vital enzyme in the body. DAO regulates the presence of histamine so it's important. And before a histamine-heavy meal, it's thought taking a supplement that boosts your DAO level can help.

We like the Ancestral Health Grass Fed Kidney – and have found their customer service very helpful. We carry it everywhere and will often take before meals to boost our DAO levels before a histamine-heavy meal. Sadly this brand is not available in the UK, however there are one or two suppliers to be found in the EU.

Some of the notable benefits of this supplement include the following:

- Is a great source of DAO enzyme.

- Reduces bloating.

- Enhances digestion and other metabolic processes in the body.

- Reduces the severity of eczema.

- Reduces the reaction a person has when ingesting high histamine foods.

We give this supplement 8 out of 10. We prefer it the Histamine Block supplement outlined below – but you may find Histamine Block works more effectively.

Vitamin C

Otherwise known as ascorbic acid, vitamin C is important in the body. In this case, it is a natural antihistamine that is easy to find. The interesting bit about this vitamin is that it is a cofactor for diamine oxidase, and also alcohol dehydrogenase. This is the final enzyme that helps in the breakdown of histamine. Whenever you are going through those exhaustive and potent symptoms, taking 1000-1500mg of vitamin C can go a long way in calming you down.

We like Thorne Vitamin C brand for their purity.

Several studies have shown the importance of this vitamin in degrading alcohol by itself. However, you should be careful about the type of vitamin C supplements you buy. Some are laced with heavy metals, which might be toxic to your body (so go Thorne or another reputable brand). Always make sure that you only get your supplements from credible sources. The best variants are organic and come from a food-based source. The phosphatidylcholine, that is often added in these supplements, also help to support the cell membranes. Indeed some say a phosphatidylcholine such as Optimal PC by Seeking Health is also an excellent idea when it comes to the regulation of histamine in the body.

Here are the benefits of Vitamin C:

- Helps to relieve a stuffy nose.

- Prevents dire symptoms of allergies and histamine.

- Helps in the digestion process, among many other metabolic processes.

- Prevents scurvy, which normally arises due to its deficiency.

- Reduces oxidative stress.

We give a good Vitamin C supplement 6 out of 10. It probably won't be a game changer but is a good part of your histamine supplement cabinet.

DAOsin and Histamine Block

Both these supplements contain DAO, the primary enzyme that degrades ingested histamine. As much as this is a great supplement, which works effectively, we don't recommend it solely for the ingredients. DAOsin and Histamine Block are specifically useful before meals and drinks, with a few minutes gap to permit absorption. It has the DAO enzyme, which is crucial to the control of histamine. And since the DAO enzyme breaks down external histamine, this supplement will help you to break down histamine found in foods. It is also great for individuals whose digestive tract is filled with histamine-producing bacteria.

So why don't we like it? All available brands in this area at the time of writing contain talc (or hydrated magnesium stearate to give it the official title). Talc is added to supplements to prevent ingredients from clumping and sticking to machinery when forming tablets, and talc as a food additive is "generally recognized as safe" by the FDA. That said, there are numerous articles online suggesting that it is not a great ingredient to be including in a supplement. Talc is not known to pose a risk of cancer when consumed from supplements. We'll leave you to do your own research on the inclusion of hydrated magnesium stearate in a supplement.

Otherwise, here are some of its key benefits:

- Helps to support inflammatory responses in the digestive tract.

- Boosts the digestion process and metabolism as a whole.

- Has an optimized stability as compared to some of the other supplements.

- It is a good source of the diamine oxidase (DAO) enzyme and users have reported excellent benefits from taking before meals.

We give this supplement 5 out of 10.

Loratadine

As a histamine intolerant patient going through a wave of painful symptoms, you may be tempted to use over the counter meds instead of seeking the right medical assistance. While this may work for you in some instances, it won't always perform as expected all the time. Therefore, thanks to evidence-based research, you might not want to lean on using so many of these OTC meds.

Loratadine is one of them, and commonly goes by the name Claritin. It is a remedy for allergies and can help you if you use it correctly. Many people who have used it before appreciate its help in terms of reducing itchiness and congestion, among many other symptoms.

Some histamine intolerant people have reported short-term improvements in using Loratadine and other OTCs, but long-term have found this approach to be less helpful.

Loratadine:

- Helps to contain allergic symptoms such as congestion, sneezing and watery eyes, among many others.

- It helps control the level of histamine in the body.

We give this 5 out of 10, but it may well be very useful for you, especially in a flare-up or on a seasonal basis.

Magnesium

Magnesium is vital for the human cells, due to several processes. For cells to use energy obtained from food, magnesium must play a role. It is also important for the build-up of muscles and the maintenance of vibrant cell walls. As if this is not enough, the mineral also helps in the maintenance of the DNA structure.

Following the major roles played by magnesium in the body, it is thought that histamine intolerance occurs partly due to its deficiency. What proves this point even further is the fact that magnesium is needed in the production of DAO – an enzyme important for histamine control, as we've already discussed.

If you don't have sufficient DAO in the body, histamine levels will increase in the body. Most of the symptoms you will go through when intolerant to histamine emanate from the release of histamine from immune cells. This is what, in turn, leads to the allergic reactions.

When you lower the blood histamine levels, you reduce these symptoms and effects. One sure way to achieve this is through the use of magnesium. On average, men should take about 300mg of magnesium while ladies should take 270mg. But we often don't get enough of this in diet.

Dr. Carolyn Dean is one of the world's top experts on Magnesium. You can find her book The Magnesium Miracle online. She's also formulated magnesium which we recommend. It's called <u>ReMag Pico-Ionic Magnesium</u> and is a great solution. You can also use some kind of magnesium chloride spray. Epsom salts also work well. The only thing you should note when using the bathing salts is that heat accelerates histamine levels (little known fact!) You could consider using lukewarm water instead of hot water, or just having an Epsom salts footbath.

Adrenal Support

Look at adrenal support and the link between that and histamine. We know we've mentioned him already but we really like Dr. Ben Lynch's Seeking Health supplements for adrenal support.

If you think your adrenals might be taxed by all this stress around the histamine, then check out his supplements, in particular Optimal Adrenal and Adrenal Cortex.

Chapter 6

THE BEST LOW-HISTAMINE LIFESTYLE PRACTICES

Before you skip this chapter, you may consider that many prominent histamine doctors regard managing stress as the key, number one ingredient in managing histamine intolerance. So now that you've seen what supplements to use for histamine control, it is equally important to look at the 'non-supplements' that might help in the same course.

Managing stress

Stress and histamine seem to go together, and it's vital that you make the lifestyle changes to compliment your diet and supplement regime.

Meditation not medication

Oh how we love meditation. It's a key part of our histamine strategy. Meditation is said to be the body's natural antihistamine. Interested? Read on.

The mind is an integral part of the body. And for this reason, it is important to maintain it at optimum levels of health. Meditation is a key part of your histamine reducing strategy. Medical experts argue that if the brain is in sound state, the body will also be alright. And this makes perfect sense because, all activities in the body run from a central command – the brain. And this includes the performance of histamine.

It helps to stabilize the mast cells. And it changes the expression from our genetics, quite literally so that one can have an epigenetic boost.

In today's prescription-filled world, many people are constantly seeking alternatives to drugs. Meditation, not medication, this is the apparent new term, loved by several people. Those who believe in meditation harness the power of the brain to come up with healing for different conditions. And this is true because healing involves the mind in many ways. Even if you take meds, you will still need the mind to be in great shape so that you can get your recovery fully. Therefore, there is a direct correlation between the mind and body, when it comes to healing.

The western world, to be more precise, has been turning to alternative methods of treatment. Meditation happens to be one major example that many have turned to for help. Today, you will see a lot of clinics offering meditation help whenever you walk down the street. However, most of these therapies are derived from the eastern world.

Meditation is slowly turning into an essential treatment tool, even for chronic cases. The only problem is that most people either overstate or underestimate its benefits. We often miss the basic healing process when we attempt to heal the body without first healing the mind.

Other benefits of meditation

Meditation helps to induce different biochemical and physiological changes in the body that reduce stress or depression. And this is good news for those suffering from histamine intolerance.

Several studies have indicated that practicing meditation can help to bring down high blood pressure and cortisol levels. Chronic stress is one of the disposing factors for histamine intolerance. When this is reduced through mindfulness meditation, your chances of going through a histareaction are brought down. Interested now?

What to do

There are different forms of meditation and it doesn't matter which one you pick. All of them are helpful towards the control of histamine intolerance. Studies have indicated that just eight hours of meditation can help you regulate HDAC and COX2 genes in the body. (That's not eight hours of meditation all at once you'll be pleased to hear.) Regulating these genes aids in mast cell stabilization. Here are some approaches you can take.

- **Mindfulness meditation** – we like the Calm app and the Waking Up app from Sam Harris. Mindfulness is the most common type of meditation used in the western world. It helps you to become aware of their current state, rather than thinking of either the past or future. This is a type of meditation that you can practice anywhere, even at home. Several research studies have pointed out the benefits of this method citing; improved memory & focus, reduced emotional tension, reduced negative emotions and improved general well being and health. It can help you drift away from your current woes, including chronic pains from the histamine attack. Which we know can be really, really hard, but every little helps.

- **Transcendental meditation** – this is a spiritual type of mediation that involves sitting still and breathing gradually. The main motive of the meditation in this instance, is to rise above the current state of being you are in.

- **Zen meditation** – it is sometimes referred to as zazen, and is a Buddhist type of meditation practice. It is not easy for you to perform this practice alone and thus; you may need to take instructions from an expert. That is why most people opt to enroll in a meditation program to get its benefits. The main goals of this practice include getting the right position and concentrating on breathing. It offers both relaxation and a renewed sense of well-being.

- **Kundalini yoga** – this type is physically engaging and thus, involves a lot of movement and deep breathing. It is also great fun and normally requires a class or teacher. However, if you have the right guide, you can learn the process at the comfort of your home. Similar to most of the other types of meditation, this practice can help to boost physical & mental agility, besides improving general body health. It can help with lower back pains, and several other chronic pains.

- **Body scan meditation** – this type of meditation can also be referred to as a progressive relaxation, or PMR. It encourages a person to look at their body carefully and trace the areas that cause a lot of tension and pain. It aims at noticing the point at which the tension starts and trying to alleviate or release it. As a practitioner, you will need to start from your feet as you go up your body. Aside from promoting relaxation and a calm spirit, progressive relaxation can also help you to improve chronic conditions such as histamine related symptoms.

- **Loving or kindness meditation** – this is otherwise known as metta meditation. It is meant to improve your moods and appreciation of life. This may help you to deal with the factors responsible for your stress levels going up. While constantly breathing in and out, you take in kindness and love towards everything in life. Like any other form of meditation, it involves repetition to make you see the positive out of misery and life's troubles. If you are particularly affected by bitterness, resentment and frustration over your histamine overload, consider using this method of meditation, but don't expect to become the Dalai Lama overnight!

Here are some final tips that will help you out while meditating:

- **Focus on the moment, rather than the results.** Since this is a process that is process-oriented, it would be great if you avoid thinking about what's in store for you at the end. Instead, wait for everything to come into place as you concentrate on the current state you are in. If you are going through a difficult time with your histamine levels, this might be the only 10 minutes in your day when you can truly be in the moment.

- **Enjoy every bit of it.** Without your mind, body and soul being in sync with the practice, it is all useless. Therefore, try and make sure that you're always looking forward to the next session.

- **Leave the judgments.** Refrain from weighing whether meditation is good or bad, right or wrong. Instead, put yourself in the current state and simply let go of everything else.

- **Appreciate the fact that you cannot be an expert on the first day.** Nobody ever starts anything as a pro. Therefore, in your initial sessions, you might find yourself drifting into thinking about tomorrow night's dinner, or something else. Don't worry when this happens. It's all part of the process.

Contrary to popular perception, meditation isn't hard to do. In fact, you can do it while comfortably seated or standing, or even walking. Like butterflies in the forest, allow the thoughts to fly in and out of the mind, freely. In case you're still stuck and don't know where and how to start the process, you can access a guided meditation book or track online (as we said earlier we recommend Calm, Waking Up apps. Glo also has excellent meditations).

Massage

Another effective non-supplement for histamine intolerance is massage. At an initial point of view, you may seem to dismiss it as a remedy for histamine intolerance. However, there is a good connection between massaging and histamine.

While a massage cannot necessarily stop histamine levels from advancing in the body, it can help with the resulting symptoms. It may be useful in dissipating the effects of the allergic reaction due to histamine. You can, therefore, get an improved tolerance level through the use of this remedy.

So, how does it work? First, you need to understand the benefits associated with the practice of massaging. It helps to boost circulation, immunity and reduces stress in the body. Several studies have shown the genuine concern that is brought about by an increased level of stress, especially in regards to histamine. While you are going through stress, you might equally increase the level of histamines in the body. There is a huge correlation between fatal health conditions and high stress levels. In brief, stress triggers ailments in the body. Massaging helps to relieve stress and put the mind at rest. So, this is the connection it has with histamine intolerance.

You can easily boost your circulation and immune system through massaging. This should especially be the case when you are at your peak of the allergic reactions and symptoms. There are different trigger points in the body for histamine. When you use massage to ease this points, you will help to tone down on the effects in due course. Since you cannot do the massage for yourself, you will need help either from a member of the family or a friend. If you cannot access either, it would be appropriate for you to sign up at your local spa. This will go a long way in solving your woes.

There are different types of massages, with distinct benefits and uses in the body.

It is important to identify with one that will have positive effects towards histamine intolerance. The most common ones are the deep tissue massage (which is the best) and the Swedish massage. While the two may be quite similar in many things, they are different from each other in various notable ways. Some of the main differences include; the area of focus, pressure applied, intended use and techniques. Both are ideal for the control of histamine intolerance, but before looking at them deeply, here are some of the other types of massages that might really help:

- **Trigger point massage.** From the name, this is a massage that is used to relive pain from the source or trigger. It is specifically great for those going through chronic pains or have other issues or conditions, like say histamine intolerance. The areas that inflict pain in your body are what are referred to as trigger points. These points can also result in pain to other body parts. By focusing on these points, this type of massage helps to alleviate the pain you feel from the body. For instance, if you are having constant pain coming from the back, you will get a back massage to help you tone down this misery. It utilizes flowing and wide strokes on the affected areas. This helps to bring a relieving and gentle effect where there is a problem or issue. It is often combined together with deep and strong pressure on the affected areas. It can work with light dressing or totally undressed on the affected part. It may take around an hour or more, depending on how chronic or serious the pain is on the body.

- **Shiatsu massage.** If you want to feel relaxed and relieve pain you're feeling from different parts of the body, this might be the right massage for you. Shiatsu is Japanese in any language, so its origin is pretty obvious. It is an ancient type of massage and has stood the test of time, in terms of its health benefits. It helps to promote a calm form and relaxation in the body. This is in addition to relieving headaches, migraines, depression, stress, anxiety and muscle tensions. It engages the whole body as opposed to a particular segment bringing you trouble. However, you may request your therapist to apply closer attention to specific areas that are most affected, in addition to the body as a whole. In this type of massage, the therapist will employ both rhythmic and pulsing pressure on the body. And so, you may not need to remove any clothing when undergoing this type of massage. It can go for an hour or more, again depending on the intensity of pain you're feeling at that moment.

- **Thai massage.** This is another great massage that we recommend, especially if you feel chronic pains and have constant stress. It helps to boost circulation of blood in the body, flexibility and energy levels. It is almost similar to yogic movement in that it utilizes the whole body. To apply firm pressure on your body, the therapist will have to use his or her fingers and palm. You may also expect your body to be twisted and turned from one position to the other. It typically goes for up to an hour, but it can take more if you request so.

- **Chair massage.** This is the simplest type of massage, which can even be done by your significant other, friend or family. All you have to do is to sit down, as per the name of the massage, and get your upper body rectified. Since it is ideal for the upper body, it is limited in terms of the areas of reach. So, it is only ideal for those who have fatigue or pain on the neck, back and shoulders. This type of massage is also the best for beginners who are just starting out the practice. Aside from reducing your fatigue, this massage can equally help you out if you want to improve your relaxation and cut down stress. It employs light pressure, or sometimes medium if the case is severe. It is best to use a custom chair for the massage, but if you don't have, any chair would be okay. It usually goes for up to 30 minutes or even less.

Now, those are the basic types of massage that will help you with your histamine intolerance symptoms. However, if you're looking to go a notch higher in massaging and use the best types that will deliver incredible results, take a look at the following two keenly:

1. **Swedish massage** – this is one of the best and most familiar techniques of massaging offered. It is common in most parlors and is what may also go by the name "classic massage." It not only aims at relaxation, but is also a remedy for muscle tension, fatigue and several other complications. It is a bit gentle when compared to deep tissue massage (which we will look at next). It is particularly helpful to those who have fatigue on their necks,

lower backs and shoulders. However, it can also work for other parts of the body. It is a bit complex than the other massages pointed out earlier, as it employs different practices. For instance, you can expect your therapist to use long strokes, kneading, joint movements and circular movements, among many others. All the methods used are targeted at stimulating your nerve endings, creating a relaxation and increasing blood flow in the body. They may also help in lymph draining. Here, you can request your therapist to either use light, medium or firm pressure, depending on how severe your pain is, or your typical preferences. You can also request them to apply more pressure on particular segments that you find more painful.

2. **Deep tissue massage** – the other type of massage that is equally very effective is deep tissue massage. It is almost identical to the Swedish massage, but goes a little deeper. It is best suited for those who have excessive and chronic pains. Some examples include athletes, those with injuries and the sick. It is especially great for those with deep lower back pain and fibromyalgia. It targets the tendons, muscles and the connective tissues. Most of the elements used during a deep tissue massage are similar to those used in a Swedish massage. The only difference is that the pressure applied is more, and this may result in pain at that particular moment. From the name, the therapist needs to access the deep tissues and thus, they would need to use excessively firm pressure on your body. But this is no cause for alarm due to their high precision and skill. It may

also include using fists, in addition to other body parts in due process. The reason why it is ideal for histamine caused symptoms, is due to the healing process. It involves releasing the contracted tissues and muscles, to increase the circulation and flow of blood. This may be useful in the reduction of inflammation. After a deep tissue massage, it is normal to experience a bit of soreness all over the body. Don't take this as a serious problem, as it typically take a week before you're good to go. In case the soreness doesn't fade away, consider going back for another session or using ice and heat treatment.

It is imperative that you get an expert, to make sure that you are having the right type of massage. Here are a few tips that can help you out when looking to use massage as a remedy for your complications:

- **Get the right massage therapist.** It is enough to visit any massage parlor, but it takes a person who knows his or her job well, for the benefits to be accrued. Therefore, it is very important to only allow a professional to work on your body. To better this experience, make sure that the therapist you choose identifies with the exact type of massaging that you pick.

- **Be open to your therapist.** If there are any specific points where you want extra attention, make sure that your therapist is aware. Conversely, if there are certain parts you don't want them to touch, feel free to point them out categorically. For example, some people would not be comfortable when the therapist touches their buttocks.

- **Warm up before the massage.** This has been stated to help a lot before a massage. Therefore, consider soaking yourself in hot water prior to the session. Most professional and advanced massage parlors have saunas and hot tubs to help you get prepared.

- **Drink plenty of water.** Hydration is very important before and after your massage experience.

- **Find which massage type works best.** Of course, the above are mere suggestions on what we think would be best for you. However, if you find a particular massage type more convenient for you, then feel free to use it throughout.

If you're a bit skeptical about starting the massage procedures, seek consultations first. You may easily get a good recommendation from your doctor, friend or family member on which parlor or service to use. One more thing to do before the massage is to make sure that the massage therapist is a fully trained and certified professional. This is important to ensure that you get the best and most credible services. If you are concerned about the cost impact, you shouldn't be scared. A typical massage session can cost anything from $50-$150 in one hour. The most expensive types of massage are the aromatherapy, prenatal and hot stone variants, which luckily you don't need. However, depending on where you choose to have your massage, even a deep tissue massage may cost you a higher quote. All in all, make sure that you don't compensate quality for price. Always choose a parlor that will deliver beneficial services by the end of your experience.

Adrenal support

Here is an interesting non-supplement method for the control of histamine intolerance. Adrenal glands are one out of the many body organs affected by histamine. When the levels of this chemical rise in the body, this leads to the inflammation of the adrenal glands. These glands produce cortisol, which is useful in creating an anti-inflammatory response in the body. Therefore, a rise in the level of histamine stresses the adrenal glands. This is what can lead to the adrenal fatigue syndrome.

Adrenal support is essential to ensure that this doesn't happen. Without sufficient cortisol to counter the effects of histamine, these glands begin to wear off. When the case becomes chronic, you will start to suffer from untold pains emanating from inflammation. This is especially true for the joints and muscles. The worst-case scenario is when all this happens and you have an increased level of stress in the body. Through therapy for the adrenal glands, you will easily contain inflammation and other symptoms arising from the rise in histamine levels. The important part is to recognize the role that is played by histamine in the adrenal glands and how to prevent it. This way, you will easily manage the condition.

Stressing the adrenal glands over time results in them burning up, due to the long-term production of cortisol. As there's no sure test for adrenal fatigue, this makes it even worse to control. You might be tempted to think that it is a normal body reaction when it really isn't. Luckily, there are a few tips to help you tone down on adrenal fatigue. Some of these tips include the following:

- Avoiding junk foods and drinks.

- Consuming less sugar, especially processed sugars.

- Using nutritional supplements – these include some vitamins and minerals such as magnesium, vitamin C and vitamin B.

Some would recommend that you take a special diet for adrenal fatigue. And this may help you to reduce the effects and make your immune system stronger.

Having known the basic histamine supplements and non-supplements, it is equally important to take a look at one of the enzymes that regulate the existence of this chemical. Therefore, read on the text to learn more about DAO enzyme.

Chapter 7

WHAT IS DAO, AND HOW CAN THIS HELP ME?

We've already spoken a little about DAO and we wanted to just go over why this is so important.

What the Dao?

Diamine oxidase, popularly abbreviated as DAO, is an enzyme in the human body. It is useful during digestion and its deficiency can cause a rise in the levels of histamine in the body. It is produced in the kidneys, intestinal lining of the digestive tract and the thymus. It helps to break down the excess histamine in the body, and that's why its deficiency causes problems.

Histamine is naturally occurring in the body and helps in different functions including digestion, in the central nervous system and in the immune system. Thus, to say that you want to get rid of this chemical compound is a fallacy – it is impossible. However, you can maintain it in optimum levels so that it doesn't affect the body through symptoms that we know you've been experiencing. If you have experienced any of the symptoms of histamine intolerance or any allergy for that matter, you do know how painful it can get.

Increasing your DAO

To regulate histamine, and prevent it from getting to uncomfortable levels, it can be a good idea to increase the levels of DAO enzyme in the body. After all, many suspect that it is the deficiency of this enzyme that often causes our intolerance in the first place. The basic explanation for this is that when the levels of DAO are low in the body, it becomes hard to metabolize and get rid of excess histamine. This then leads to the rising of histamine levels, which is responsible for the ugly symptoms that meant you bought this book in the first place.

Several factors can cause the deficiency of DAO in the body. It is still those same factors that may trigger the overproduction of histamine. Alcohol use, intestinal bacteria and particular meds might be the first place to look. They are some of the risk factors for the depletion of DAO and increase in the levels of histamine.

The scientific relationship between DAO and histamine is still not understood well. We just know there are links between DAO deficiency and the accelerators of histamine production.

Supplements

When you have a deficiency of DAO, it is appropriate to use different supplements to boost its presence. We spoke about these in the supplements chapter, and as with everything in the world of histamine intolerance, it's worth playing around with these supplements to discover what works for you.

Such supplements (the grass-fed Kidney and the DAOsin) also help to break down histamine getting into your system through other avenues like foods and drinks. You know what it's like, you've eaten something in a restaurant, only to find out later that it was way high in histamine. DAO supplements can help you with this. The key word is sometimes. It won't help everyone, depending on what type of histamine intolerance you have.

DAO can be effective for histamine control both inside the body and outside. It mainly functions inside the kidneys and thymus as stated earlier. It works together with histamine N-methyl transferase, abbreviated as HNMT. Both of these enzymes help to break down histamine when it is in excess. The excess histamine is what is also known as the endogenous histamine. It is released from the mast cells due to different reasons including; trauma, infections, food induction, allergies, chronic inflammation and many other disorders.

DAO mixes with food going through the digestive tract. It helps to break it down to prevent histamine dominance inside the body. Also, as the enzyme encounters histamine in the food, it attempts to break it down. Almost all of the endogenous histamine molecules are broken down when DAO enzyme exists in good proportion. But when it is deficient, this is where the problem starts.

What happens if you go low?

You may need to observe a stricter version of the diets in this book when your levels of DAO enzyme in the body go low.

Often people assume two things – that taking DAO supplements cure histamine, and that these supplements help to increase the level of DAO produced by the body. Unfortunately, neither is true. These supplements can only ensure that the normal amount of DAO enzyme is produced, and not any extra.

Also, they only reduce the amount of histamine getting into the body and they do not cure your histamine intolerance. So DAO supplements can work, but they're not the magic pill (if only…)

Important: DAO deficiency is not always the cause of histamine spikes. There are other factors that cause histamine to get out of control. However, you still might want to make sure that you have sufficient DAO enzyme, just in case this is the reason. After all, it is equally an important enzyme that performs several roles in the body.

As briefly mentioned above, a person's genetics may play a role in their histamine intolerance condition. Wondering how? Read on the text to find out fascinating information you probably didn't know before.

Chapter 8

How do my genetics play a role in histamine intolerance?

Okay, get ready to get technical.

Genes are important, especially when it comes to histamine. However if you are new to Histamine Intolerance you may want to come back to this section once you've covered off more of the 'low-hanging fruit' that will help you to get faster results.

<u>Is histamine intolerance hereditary?</u>

You want to get a 23andme test (or other provider) to take a look at your gene profile at this point, to understand where you are at in terms of potential genetics and histamine.

Here are some of the gene mutations (we don't like that word, but it's the word that the community seem to have settled on) that have an impact on histamine intolerance.

PEMT

This is a gene that encodes and converts the phosphatidylethanolamine into phosphatidylcholine. It is fully known scientifically as phosphatidylethanolamine N-methyltransferase. Yep, long name.

It does this in the liver and the chemical it produces is vital in the cell membranes. It helps to stabilize these membranes and maintain them under normal or healthy conditions.

MAO

This is a gene that needs a cofactor of B2. The gene is also polymorphic and a bit slower in men than in women. Thus, you can see men suffering from histamine intolerance and being more vulnerable than women. This gene not only helps to regulate histamine levels in the body, but also helps to contain tyramines and catecholamines. These catecholamines are what are termed as stress neurotransmitters. Therefore, we can also claim that depression, anxiety and stress may be genetic – a case for another day. MAO gene equally helps to reduce migraines and headaches through the induction of riboflavin.

COMT

Aside from breaking down estrogen, this gene also helps to break the stress neurotransmitters. When your estrogen levels and stress neurotransmitters are high, chances are that your histamine levels will also shoot up. Therefore, this gene is quite necessary in the body – its deficiency can lead to the dominance of histamine.

DAO

This is no longer new to you as we have handled it severally. However, its importance cannot be overemphasized. This gene requires copper as its cofactor to function optimally. Equally, it is polymorphic just like the MAO gene. It specifically helps to tone down extracellular histamine. This is the histamine resulting from food and bacteria. Therefore, when you have a variation in this gene, you might find it difficult eating certain foods and drinks. Also, you might need to eat everything fresh or from the freezer. There should be no chance for bacteria to develop. It will also necessitate you to take constant DAO enzyme supplements to help you reduce histamine inside the body. Thus, this is the most sensitive gene because humans cannot survive without food and need to eat. It limits what you can eat and what you can't.

MTHFR

This is a gene that is useful in regulating methylation. Opposed to DAO, it helps to reduce intracellular histamine. Its cofactor for an optimal performance is B2.

HNMT

This is yet another great gene that works hand in hand with its DAO counterpart. It helps in the production of HNMT enzyme. It needs SAMe as a cofactor to function optimally. Like the MTHFR gene, it cuts down on intracellular histamine. Aside from all that, it is polymorphic.

Besides all that, methylation is impacted to a great extent. Stressing methylation is one sure way to histamine intolerance – no doubt about that. This will force your histamine bucket to overfill since your body will be handling several things at the same time. Reducing stress is, thus, a good thing to do both for your well-being and body. Since it is an integral factor for histamine intolerance, you can balance stress through the following ways:

- Sleep. Just having a rest of mind and body is enough to deal with stress. Your inability to sleep well may affect your stress levels. Insomnia often causes depression and stress in the body. Make sure that you get sufficient hours to rest every day, no matter the schedule you have.

- Breathing. This might sound obvious or stupid but yes, are you correctly breathing? A constant flow of air in and out of the body is vital if you want to evade stress. And mindfulness meditation can help you do this effectively. You need constant belly air whenever possible.

- Oxygenation. Differentiate this from breathing as it entails having a good aeration inside your room. You need to get rid of stuffy air and stale essence that may cause you stress.

- Eating. Food is important for everything, including the prevention of stress in the body. Several nutrients are needed to prevent the mind from getting depressed. Therefore, it is not just enough to eat, but to eat a balanced diet.

- Constant exercise. Aerobic and anaerobic exercises are key to living a healthy life free of stress. Depending on the schedule you hold, you can allocate a few hours for exercises in a day. This will go a long way in salvaging your situation.

The above is particularly important when your genes suggest a predisposition to histamine spikes. When you have the wrong diet, lifestyle, supplements or environment, there is a high chance your histamine levels can increase. *This is further worsened if you have a gene deficiency that predisposes you to histamine intolerance, and makes the above lifestyle changes all the more important.*

Chapter 9

HOW TO MEASURE MY PERSONAL HISTAMINE LEVELS

As we've already looked at, there are some tests out there for histamine intolerance. However none are particularly conclusive. Here's something we love though, in terms of your own histamine levels, and a kind-of A/B split testing for your own histamine wellness.

Histamine and heart rate.

It is well-documented that histamine intolerance can have an adverse effect on our heart rate. And for many people, it produces a spiking heart rate. It certainly does for us. In other words, when you eat more histamine-rich food than your body can handle, your heart rate goes up.

It's surprisingly difficult to test for histamine intolerance. However, we found a far more effective way of testing histamine levels. And that is to use a simple activity tracker, of which there are many on the market and analyze your heart rate and heart rate variability.

Track your heart rate at home

We found, the more that we eat a low-histamine diet and cut out those avocados, the chocolates, the leftovers and even the tomatoes as well, and the more that we take the supplements that are good for us – the probiotics that are histamine friendly, the quercetin, the grass fed kidney and so on. When we do those things, we've noticed that our overnight heart rate comes down quite considerably. And on the days when we slip up and have a glass of red wine or eat some leftovers, our heart rate shoots up.

Why is this a great hack? Because by tracking your heart rate, you can now start to discover the foods that you're not sure about. Forget reading the online guides to histamine intolerance that may or may not apply to you. You're now starting to compile your very own personalized histamine list.

Low Histamine Secret Sauce!

How does it work?

Here's an example. You're not sure whether chocolate boosts your histamine levels to the extent that it makes you feel bad? You wear an activity tracker and establish a baseline for your heart rate. You then eat the suspect food – i.e. chocolate. You suspect that there may be an issue, but you're not sure. Eat some chocolate and check your overnight heart rate. If it has spiked, bingo, you have a problem.

Which tracker to use?

Low Histamine Secret Sauce!

This is the second secret sauce alert in this chapter. Our favorite tracker is the Oura ring, produced by a Finnish company, and now based mostly in the United States. It's a small ring that you can wear on any finger or indeed thumb. And it could be a big part of our recovery. This measures plenty of metrics including; heart rate, heart rate variability, total sleep/deep sleep, body temperature and respiratory rate. Also measured is your activity and steps, which is the kind of thing that most activity trackers measure. With the Oura ring, we can tell the next day when we've eaten a histamine-heavy meal. And it is quite revealing.

Over the course of days, weeks and months, you can start to track your histamine levels and do what works. There are other trackers that also work really well.

Garmin make some quite sophisticated heart rate and heart rate variability (HRV) trackers. Our favorite is the Oura ring, because it is so small, it doesn't have a display and you can put it into airplane mode. Therefore, switching off the electromagnetic fields, associated with Bluetooth or Wi-Fi.

But if you want to go for a wristwatch, the best Garmins to purchase for heart rate and heart rate variability (HRV), are the Garmin 945, the Garmin Fenix 5 or the Garmin Vivo Smart 3. Other Garmin watches are not necessarily guaranteed to give you heart rate variability, which is really important. Garmin can also be put into airplane mode by switching Bluetooth off on the device.

Garmin have a feature called Stress Index, which might help you a lot with your histamine knowledge, and your personalized histamine recommendations. The Apple Watch also measures heart rate and heart rate variability and many have found this an effective tracker, particularly for HRV. We will leave you to look into this further.

But the Oura Ring is still our favourite. NB – make sure you get the right size. They have a free sizing kit if like us you're not used to wearing rings. Our first Oura

Ring unfortunately got lost on day two – absolutely gutted. Now we were it on the thumb and it's nice and cosy. We even get comments on how cool it looks (though we're not convinced)

<u>Wait, how much?</u>

Yes, some of these options are expensive. We know that. But many of these histamine tests are very inconclusive. They depend on the time of day, what you ate the night before and they are not that accurate anyway. It's difficult because most doctors don't see histamine intolerance as a problem. The medical community and those in the media sometimes, poorly understand it. And that's why we have to come up with our own solutions.

As renowned biohacker Ben Greenfield says, (and we're paraphrasing here); yes it costs a lot to look after your health in this way, but it costs a lot more if you end up in hospital because you *haven't* looked after your health.

Of course, if this particular tracking histahack costs too much for you at the moment, there are plenty of other hacks and practices in this book that don't cost anything. There is also a useful app called EliteHRV that tracks your heart rate and heart rate variability. We have found it's not particularly accurate and requires a lot of time sitting with your thumb attached to a phone, but is a good free solution. Available on iPhone and Android.

We hope that this tracking solution may provide some of the most effective 'secret sauce' in your histamine intolerance detective work. It has for us. Using this simple technology that has never been available before, the activity trackers and measuring your heart rate and heart rate variability can give you some answers around histamine.

Chapter 10

WHY DOESN'T MY DOCTOR KNOW ABOUT HISTAMINE INTOLERANCE?

What's up Doc?

Histamine intolerance is certainly not a key part of the medical syllabus, though we are hugely grateful for the numerous enlightened and open-minded medical practitioners who've helped us along the way.

As we've discovered, histamine intolerance is very tough to test for. And this is one of the reasons why most doctors fail to diagnose it early enough, or on the initial visit by the patient.

Most of its signs and symptoms are similar to those of many other mainstream diseases and complications. When a doctor only has 10 minutes to talk to you, hear your story and your symptoms and make a diagnosis, as we know it's often just not going to happen straightaway. It may take deeper research for an individual to unearth histamine intolerance.

So, in short, your frequent visits to a medical facility may prove futile for the first few attempts. The doctor may fail to tell you what's going on, and you can't really blame them (as I said we love our Doc, we just want them to help us through this.)

Histamine intolerance is complex and is thus, not easy to diagnose. Our research has shown that numerous patients get misdiagnosed with other allergies and ailments, only to discover in the end, that it was histamine all along.

Symptoms worsening over time

The other reason why diagnosis poses a challenge is because of the build-up of symptoms over time.

The conventional tests that were used to diagnose allergies, are not always effective for histamine intolerance. These are the likes of ELISA IgE antibody blood tests and skin prick tests. These can provide clues, but aren't conclusive.

The sure way to diagnose the case, that is being used to date, is by attempting the histamine-free diet in this book, the supplements and the lifestyle programs and seeing if you start to improve. If you do, then you know, and so in some ways you can arrive at your diagnosis before you doctor.

It's tough for your Doc

Before arriving at the diagnosis of histamine intolerance, your doctor will have to first rule out everything else, literally. *All* the possible diseases have to be cleared before arriving at histamine intolerance – pretty amazing, huh? So perhaps it's understandable you aren't going to walk out of the surgery with a conclusive diagnosis.

Elimination diet and other possible ways to diagnose

Your physician may equally encourage you to try out elimination as a way to discover if you are suffering from the disorder. He or she may instruct that you avoid certain foods and drinks for a given period, say 15-30 days. This will need you to reintroduce these foods once again after the set time so that the reactions are visible once again.

Thanks to advancements in medicine, a new test for the DAO enzyme deficiency has emerged recently. It involves taking a blood sample from you and trying to analyze for any possible traces of the deficiency.

Confusingly, most symptoms from the disorder are similar to other food allergies and lactose intolerance or malabsorption of fructose. They are also a little bit similar to those of the celiac disease, so the elimination test and the DAO enzyme deficiency tests can provide clues for your Doc.

Dear Diary, I think I have histamine intolerance

When you start to talk about your histamine intolerance with a doctor, or health practitioner, you will have to open up about your lifestyle, nutritional habits, and symptoms.

Therefore, it may be a good idea for you to have a symptom diary prior to visiting the doctor. If you suspect that what you're going through is histamine intolerance, record everything you feel. Leave nothing to chance, as even the slightest symptom will help in the diagnosis.

Moreover, if you already have a clue on which foods might be worsening your case, then you can also keep a record of them for the doctor. Besides, pundits in the medicine niche have also argued that medication is a massive contributor to how someone feels when faced with histamine intolerance. Thus, it is essential to tell the doctor all the meds you've been taking. And for better results, you can keep all your prior medical reports and prescriptions ready. You will, later on, learn that some medicines trigger histamine levels to rise. Others may also force the body to produce its histamine.

Your doctor first has to rule out the mainstream diseases, before focusing on allergies, food intolerances, and mastocytosis. Then they might suggest an elimination diet.

- **Elimination diet.** You will be given a symptom diary, and as stated earlier, will be required to avoid certain foods. You will record whether or not the symptoms you have been facing stop. Later on, you will again start eating the same foods and drinking the same drinks then be watchful over the symptoms. If they reappear, then this will mean that you might have the disorder. All symptoms should be strictly recorded to make it easier for the doctor to make his or her judgment.

Of course, you could start with a low-histamine diet right now by continuing with the program in this book.

After the elimination test, your Doc can suggest the provocation test if doubts are still present. This is the next step once you're back to the medical facility, with results from the elimination diet. It is mostly the final test conducted on a patient. The downside of this test is that there might be a risk of anaphylactic shock. Therefore, it should only be **STRICTLY** carried out under **MEDICAL SUPERVISION** from a qualified professional.

Diagnosis

As you are learning, you might never get an official medical diagnosis of histamine intolerance. Many doctors are still learning about the debilitating effects of histamine intolerance. But many do know all about it, and you might have one of the good ones!

After your diagnosis, the doctor will give the way forward that you will need to follow to the latter. This may involve changing your lifestyle entirely and making massive diet changes. For more on this, read on the book in the following chapters.

In conclusion, a histamine intolerance diagnosis is a possibility, but don't keep your hopes high. It is a procedural type of diagnosis that will go on for weeks, and even months before the final results emerge. Thus, you need to be patient and dedicated. You must follow all the guidelines given, especially for the elimination diet.

Chapter 11

FIVE WAYS TO REDUCE MY HISTAMINE BUCKET RIGHT NOW!

Whatever you're going through, it's important to note that there's no substitute for medical advice. Please seek medical advice for your histamine symptoms. If your histamine bucket is overflowing right now, we have huge sympathy for you. We've been there. We have put this handy and quick guide together so you can reduce your histamine bucket right now:

1. TAKE SUPPLEMENTS

This includes:

- Loratadine (over the counter medication),

- HistaminX (supplement sold by Seeking health – contains a number of natural compounds),

- ProBiota HistaminX

- Quercetin (natural compound proven to reduce histamine levels in the body - BioCare),

- Pycnogenol (made from tree bark),

- Surthrival Colostrum (grass fed tablets – great for immunity and general health)

- Ancestral Health Grass Fed Kidney to increase your DAO levels (Ancestral Health supplements sell a brilliant version of this, and this has helped us tremendously). In fact, we take these supplements before meals, around 20-30 minutes before the meal. And that helps our DAO levels.

- Vitamin C (Thorne or Seeking Health liposomal)

As always, check with your doctor before taking any new supplements, but these work for us. If you are in an emergency situation, please go to the emergency room or the hospital, or your doctor.

2. MEDITATION

We get it. It is frustrating to be going through a histamine episode, feeling dreadful and someone suggesting, "hey why don't you sit with your legs crossed in a Om position, and try to just chill out."

But it really does work. We like meditating in front of an infrared light (we recommend Joovv), which can help with all sorts of things, but seems to just be very relaxing. Y

Also use Binaural Beats, which you can purchase as a cheap app. This plays a slightly different tone in each ear, to take you into different brain wave states to take you from that high beat state that you might be in at the moment into alpha then theta, then delta – which are the states associated with deep relaxation. We know this isn't easy when the bucket is overflowing, but it really does help.

3. MAGNESIUM

You might also want to get involved with magnesium. We like ionic liquid magnesium supplements, but we also love magnesium chloride spray, which is a really easy way to absorb magnesium transdermally and quickly. As detailed elsewhere, magnesium can help with histamine levels.

Dr. Carolyn Dean is one of the world's greatest experts on Magnesium and you can find her book The Magnesium Miracle online.

4. ADRENAL SUPPORT

Look at adrenal support. And we really like Dr. Ben Lynch's Seeking Health supplements for adrenal support – Optimal Adrenal and Adrenal Cortex.

If you think your adrenals might be taxed by all this stress around the histamine, then check out his adrenal supplements. Good luck with reducing the bucket, it will go down.

5. COCONUT CHARCOAL

If your symptoms are gut related, we have found that activated coconut charcoal seems to work particularly well, in an immediate reduction of the symptoms. It works by absorbing all the toxins in the gut.

Bulletproof make an excellent version of this, and we take it everywhere.

Low Histamine Secret Sauce!

This is the final secret sauce moment in the book, and at first glance it may seem a strange one. But read on.

Thankfully, charcoal tablets are now a last resort for us, but once upon a time, we relied on them regularly. *If you suffer specifically from gut-related histamine symptoms, charcoal may well be your friend.* Binders are important, and a gentle coconut charcoal like the bulletproof charcoal may be just the thing for you.

Make sure you drink plenty of water when you take charcoal tablets as they can dehydrate you. But if your issues are gut related, you may find this really helps – sometimes working in about ten minutes.

Remember, charcoal tablets are something to carry around in your bag, ready to take when the bucket overflows. They are like firefighters in the gut, going in to rescue your gut and put out the histamine fire. They may not be the long-term solution to your histamine issues, but if they work as well for you as they do for us, you'll get a tremendous amount of instant relief from them.

Chapter 12

THE FUTURE: LIVING A HAPPY LOW-HISTAMINE LIFE

Uh – is there histamine in that?

Ultimately, histamine intolerance is a frustrating condition. Try going around to your friends for dinner or to a restaurant, and asking them to cook you a low histamine dish. They will look at you blankly and think you're making it up. What the hell is this guy talking about? – they will think.

But now, you know. You know that you are not alone. You know that there are many other people who have gone through similar circumstances to that which you are living through now. And that is why we have compiled this book.

Resources

The great thing is that there are some brilliant resources out there. The Histamine Intolerance Awareness Group is a closed Facebook group, where hundreds of supportive messages are posted a day, and you can ask any question. Want to know if onions bring you out in hives? Post in this group. Want to know if saunas are good or bad for histamine intolerance? Post in this group. There are a number of other great resources out there.

As discussed we find the Swiss Interest Group Histamine Intolerance or SIGHI in abbreviation, to have the best and most comprehensive food compatibility list for histamine. And it may well be worth downloading this one to your phone. They rank each food with compatibility, histamine levels, liberators and blockers. In other words, they'll tell you how high the histamine level is in the food. Whether it liberates histamine, or blocks histamine or has any other histamine effects. And you can pick almost any food, and it will be on here, with some remarks where appropriate as well.

<u>Parting thoughts</u>

In some ways, having histamine intolerance is a gift, though you may not feel like it at the moment. Here's how we have brightsided our condition:

> *Histamine Intolerance forces you to look at every aspect of your health and well-being.*

And hopefully, twenty years down the line, you'll be living a whole lot healthier than you would have been had you not had histamine intolerance. You will have thought much more deeply about your sleep, your meditation, your exercise, your diet, your supplementary intake and your whole lifestyle than you ever would have – and that is a gift.

Good luck, and we wish you a happy low-histamine lifestyle, long into the future.

Made in the
USA
Columbia, SC